Peripheral Neuropathy for Diabetics

Your Guide to Taking Control by Reversing Diabetic Neuropathy and Feeling Better

Alex Locklear

<u>Table of content:</u>

Introduction:

How Peripheral Neuropathy and Diabetes Are Related and Affect Each Other

Perhaps you or someone you care about has been told they have diabetes and has also heard of peripheral neuropathy. This condition, which is often a result of diabetes, can be painful and cause worry. But knowing things gives you power. You can take charge of your health and well-being if you know about peripheral neuropathy, how it affects your life, and how it is linked to diabetes. Getting this information is the first thing you need to do to thrive.

What does peripheral neuropathy mean?

This is a disease that impacts the nerves that are not in your brain or spinal cord. It is part of the peripheral nervous system. The nerves in your body are like a huge web of lines that connect your brain and spinal cord to the rest of your body. They are in charge of everything, from how you move and feel to how your cells work. If these nerves get hurt, it can cause a lot of different symptoms, from tingling and stiffness to pain and muscle weakness.

How diabetes and peripheral neuropathy are linked There are a lot of different ways that diabetes and peripheral neuropathy are connected. Diabetes is a long-term disease where your blood sugar levels are too high. Over time, it can hurt your nerves. Most of the time, this damage happens slowly and may not be seen at first. This is why it's so important to see your doctor regularly for early diagnosis and treatment.

In more than one way, having high blood sugar can hurt your feelings. It can hurt the blood vessels that bring oxygen and food to your nerves, which can damage them. It can also hurt nerves directly by making it hard for them to send and receive messages. Diabetes can also cause inflammation, which can hurt nerves even more.

What Peripheral Neuropathy Does to Your Life

Peripheral neuropathy can make your daily life very hard. The symptoms may be mild to serious, and they may make it hard for you to do normal things. When your hands and feet feel numb and tingly, it can be hard to hold things, walk, or even feel changes in temperature. Pain can be constant or come and go, and it can be anything from mild discomfort to serious agony. It can be hard to move your arms, keep your balance, and do everyday things when your muscles are weak.

In addition to the physical signs, peripheral neuropathy can also affect a person's mood and mental health. Being in pain and limited all the time can make people angry, anxious, and even depressed. Don't forget that you're not on this trip by yourself. Around the world, millions of people live with peripheral neuropathy. You can deal with your symptoms and keep living a full life if you get the right help and tools.

How to Do Well While Living with Peripheral Neuropathy

Even though peripheral neuropathy can be hard, it doesn't have to control your life. You can better your quality of life and control your symptoms by learning about your condition, working closely with your healthcare team, and making the changes to your lifestyle that are needed. This journey isn't just about dealing with a disease; it's also about doing well in spite of it.

In the next few chapters, we'll talk more about the different kinds of peripheral neuropathy, the different kinds of treatments that are available, and useful ways to deal with your symptoms. We will also talk about how a good lifestyle, emotional health, and the support of your community can help you do well with peripheral neuropathy.

Don't forget that this is your journey. Conditions don't make you who you are. You can not only live with peripheral neuropathy but also do well despite it if you know what to do, are strong, and get the right help. We should start this trip together.

Stepping up and taking charge of your health and well-being

It can be hard to deal with diabetes and nerve neuropathy. It's hard to deal with the tingling, weakness, and pain. But there is good news: you can do something. As it turns out, you have a lot of power to change your health and well-being. You can step into that power with the help of this lesson.

How Knowledge Can Help You

To be empowered, you must first know what you're doing. You can make better choices if you know more about peripheral neuropathy, diabetes, and how they affect each other. Read books, articles, and sources you can trust. Talk to your doctor, nurses, and other people who work in health care. Question a lot and don't be afraid to do it. Don't forget that information isn't just power; it's also trust.

Putting together your healthcare team

Your health care team has you as their boss. It's your life, your health, and your body. You don't have to do it by yourself, though. Put together a group of skilled and helpful professionals who can help you on your upcoming journey. A neurologist, a podiatrist, a diabetes educator, a registered dietitian, and maybe even a mental health worker could be in this group. Work together with your medical staff. Tell us about your hopes, worries, and thoughts. Take an active role in your care. Don't forget that it's a relationship. There is one goal that you and your healthcare team are working toward: your health and well-being.

How You Live Is Medicine

Things like what you eat, how much you move, and how well you sleep are not just choices you make for yourself. They are strong tools that can have a big effect on your health and well-being.

Having a healthy diet is important for managing diabetes and can also help keep your brain healthy. Eat lots of fruits, veggies, whole grains, lean protein, and other foods that have not been processed. Cut back on refined carbs, added sugar, and saturated fat.

Another important tool is regular physical exercise. It

lowers pain, improves circulation, keeps blood sugar in check, and makes you feel better. It's important to make time for things you enjoy, like walks, swimming, dancing, and gardening.

Your body needs sleep to rest and heal. Aim to get at least 7-8 hours of good sleep every night. If you can't sleep, you should see a doctor. There are many things you can do, from taking medicine to learning how to relax, to help you sleep better.

How living with neuropathy makes you feel

Not only is living with peripheral neuropathy hard on the body, it's also hard on the emotions. It's okay to be upset, angry, sad, or even depressed. Be honest about how you feel. Seek help from friends, family, or a support group. Connecting with other people and talking about your experiences can be very powerful.

How Thinking Positively Can Help You

How you think matters. Having a good attitude can make a big difference in your health and happiness. Be aware, show gratitude, and be kind to yourself. Think about what you can do instead of what you can't. No matter how small, celebrate your wins. Don't forget that every day is a chance to do well.

Don't forget that this is your journey. You're not by yourself, and you can do something. You can take care of your health and well-being and live a full and vibrant life with peripheral neuropathy if you know what to do, get help, and have the right tools.

Chapter 1: Decoding Neuropathy: Types, Causes, and Symptoms

Diabetic Neuropathy: A Closer Look

Millions of people around the world have diabetes, which is a long-term disease. Several things can go wrong because of it. One of these problems is diabetic neuropathy, which is nerve loss that only happens to people with diabetes. It's important to understand this sickness so that you can live a healthy and happy life, even if it sounds scary. This part goes into more depth about diabetic neuropathy, including what it looks like and how it might be treated.

What does neuropathy caused by diabetes mean?

Nerve damage from having high blood sugar for a long time is what diabetes neuropathy is all about. In different parts of the body, this damage leads to different kinds of neuropathy. Peripheral neuropathy makes nerves in the hands and feet more likely to bother people. Mostly, it feels like tingly, being stiff, being in pain, or burning.

How does diabetes hurt nerves?

Some things may play a role in how neuropathy is caused by diabetes, but no one knows for sure. When your blood sugar is too high, it can damage the blood vessels that bring nutrients to your nerves. This can weaken them. Having high blood sugar can also change chemicals in the body in ways that hurt nerves. Over time, this harm can add up and cause nerve pain.

Different Ways Diabetes Neuropathy Looks

Diabetic neuropathy shows up in different ways for different people. Different nerves can cause it to show up in different ways. Let me talk about the different kinds with you:

You can get this kind of neuropathy in your hands and feet the most. It's possible for the pain and loss of feeling to be very bad, or they can be mild, like tingly and numbness.

2. Autonomic neuropathy: This kind affects the nerves that manage breathing, heart rate, and urine control. People who have it may feel dizzy or weak, have stomach problems, and need to go to the bathroom more than once.

The muscles in the knees, thighs, and hips are most often affected by this type, which is less common. It hurts, makes you weak, and makes it hard to move. 4. Focal neuropathy: This type only affects one nerve and can suddenly weaken a muscle or group of muscles.

How to Read the Signs

To take care of diabetic neuropathy well, it is very important to find it early. You can fix the problem and keep it from getting worse if you know what the signs are.
The following are some common signs of peripheral neuropathy:
Pain in the feet or hands that feels like it's on fire Touch sensitivity, weak muscles, and trouble walking or standing are some of the signs.

If you have autonomic neuropathy, you might feel dizzy or faint when you stand up, have stomach problems like diarrhea or constipation, leak urine, have trouble getting or keeping an erection, or have trouble controlling your body temperature.

If you have any of these signs, you should see your doctor right away to get a full analysis. If you get help and are diagnosed early, things will get better and your life will be better in general.

How to deal with diabetic neuropathy and take charge of your life

There is no fix for diabetic neuropathy, but there are many ways to deal with the symptoms, stay healthy, and feel better overall. These things are possible:

1. Keeping blood sugar in check: One important part of handling diabetes neuropathy is keeping blood sugar levels at a healthy level. Getting enough

exercise, eating well, and taking your medicines as directed are all important parts of this.

2. Medicines: Different medicines can help ease pain and other signs of neuropathy. Medicines like gabapentin and pregabalin that you get from your doctor, over-the-counter pain killers, and creams or patches that you put on your skin are some of these.

3. Making changes to how you live: Being healthy can make a big difference in how well you deal with neuropathy. To do this, they need to stay at a healthy weight, stop smoking, drink less alcohol, and make sure they get enough sleep.

4. Physical therapy: The exercises in physical therapy can make you stronger, more steady, and better coordinated. This can make you less likely to trip and hurt yourself.

5. Different kinds of therapy: Alternative therapies, such as acupuncture, massage, or ways to relax, may help some people feel better.

A Journey of Hope and Strength

Diabetes can make your nerves hurt, but it doesn't have to be your life. Know what's going on, take steps to control it, and keep a positive mood. This will help you get through hard times and do well. Remember that you're not on this trip by yourself. You can ask your doctors, family, and friends for help. Diabetes can cause nerve pain, but you can deal with it and still enjoy life with your partner.

The following are some other types of peripheral neuropathy: Also Diabetes

Diabetes is one reason why peripheral neuropathy happens, but it's not the only one. Learn more about the different types of neuropathy to get a better idea of how healthy your nerves are. Here are some more ways that these important lines of communication can be broken.

When the defense system isn't working right: autoimmune nerve damage

It's the body's job to protect us, but sometimes it fights its own nerves by mistake. Autoimmune neuropathy is the name for this kind of nerve damage. Guillain-Barré syndrome (GBS) and chronic inflammatory demyelinating polyneuropathy (CIDP) are two diseases in this group. People with GBS often feel weak and tingly all of a sudden. The signs start in the hands and feet and can spread quickly. Sometimes the signs of CIDP are the same, but they happen more slowly, over weeks or months.

Though getting these findings can be scary, it's good to know that there are ways to help. With quick medical care, many people with autoimmune neuropathies can keep their symptoms under control and live full lives. It is very important to find it early and work closely with your healthcare team to make a treatment plan.

Toxins and Medicines: A Danger You Can't See These days, we come across many things, and some of them may make us feel bad. Lead, mercury, and some drugs can all cause neuropathy. Heavy metals like lead and mercury can also do it. Plus, it is known that having too much alcohol can make nerve damage more likely.

Neuropathy can often be stopped from getting worse or even made better by stopping the drug that causes it. Don't be afraid to tell your doctor if you think a drug or something in the environment is making your worry worse. They can help you figure out what might be causing your symptoms and change your treatment plan if necessary.

Rare, but real, are neuropathies that run in families. Genetics can also lead to peripheral neuropathy, but it doesn't happen very often. Nerve diseases, like Charcot-Marie-Tooth, are passed down from parent to child. Most people who have these conditions get them in their teens or early 20s. Over time, they weaken muscles and make people lose their minds.

Even though there is no fix for inherited neuropathies, keeping busy and taking care of your symptoms can make a big difference in your quality of life. Physical therapy, occupational therapy, and assistive equipment can help people stay on their own and do the things they enjoy. Another thing is that research into new therapies is still going on. This gives people hope for future therapies.

Not getting enough vitamins and brain health

Food that is good for you and balanced is good for your brain and every other part of your body. Vitamins like B12 are very important for keeping your brain healthy. Nerve damage can happen if you don't get enough of these nutrients, or it can get worse if you already have it.

For the most part, it's easy to fix food deficiencies. If you don't have enough minerals or vitamins in your blood, an easy test can tell you. This can be fixed with vitamins or changes to the food, which will help the nerves stay healthy. So we know that even small changes can make a big difference in our lives. The Way Forward: Being Smart Gives You Power Keep in mind that your experience is unique, even though this chapter talks about different types of peripheral neuropathy. The type of treatment you can get and how well you will do will depend on what caused your neuropathy. But if you know what you're doing, you can look after your health and pick wise things.

Remember that you're not on this trip by yourself. This book and the help of your medical team can help you get through the hard parts of peripheral neuropathy and do well. Continue to learn and ask questions. The most important thing is to keep believing in yourself. Your strength and toughness are your best traits.

Learn how to spot the first signs of peripheral neuropathy. One of the most important things we can do on our trip is this. It gives us power because it lets us move faster instead of later. To be a good manager and make our lives better, don't forget that early finding is key.

Here are some of the most common early symptoms and signs. Often, the first sign of neuropathy is a small change in how you feel, like pins and needles. You might not want to think about that, but it's a very important early sign. If you have this, it generally starts in your feet and moves up to your legs over time. Sometimes it can happen in your arms and hands too. You need to pay attention to it right away because it's like a slow tide rising.

Pain could be the next thing that happens. This pain can be dull and burning or sharp and stabbing. Some say it feels like an electric shock, while others say it's like a constant pain that won't go away. When you touch something, even something as light as a bedsheet, this pain can start. It can also happen by itself.

Feeling tingly, numb, or in pain are not the only early signs you should be aware of. Your feet or hands might not be able to feel changes in temperature as well, or it may be hard for you to walk without losing your balance. Some people feel like their muscles are weakening, mostly in their legs and feet. Others may notice that they can't move around as well.

Remember that these early signs and symptoms can look very different for everyone. At first, they may be small and come and go, which makes it easy to miss them or think they are just a part of getting older. But it's important to pay attention to what your body is telling you and see a doctor if anything changes.

"Why is it so important to see these early signs?" comes to mind. Find out how peripheral neuropathy works to find the answer. This situation can get worse and cause more serious symptoms and problems if you don't fix it. It is often possible to stop a disease from getting worse with early detection and treatment. These steps can also help people deal with their symptoms.

Think of a yard. It's not hard to get rid of weeds if we get them when they are just sprouts. If we wait until the plant is fully grown and has deep roots, it will be much harder to get rid of. The same is true for nerve neuropathy. If we find it early, we have more options for how to treat and care for it.

What do we mean when we talk about getting help early? To begin with, it means getting checked out by your doctor. Your medical background may be looked at, and you may have some tests, such as an electromyogram or a nerve conduction study.

Once they know what's wrong, your doctor can help you make a clear plan for your care. Pain killers or other medicines, changes to your lifestyle like eating better and being more active, and sometimes treatments like physical or occupational therapy could be part of this.

Remember that knowledge is power. If we know the early warning signs and symptoms of peripheral neuropathy, we can take charge of our health and well-being. It's important to get help early on if you want to deal with this issue and live a full, busy life.

Pay attention to your body. Pay attention to the tingling, numbness, and pain that are happening in the background. If you see any changes, don't be afraid to call your doctor. We can get through this and live a good life even though we have peripheral neuropathy if we work together.

Chapter 2: Managing Pain and Discomfort

Medications for Pain Relief: Pros and Cons

Living with peripheral neuropathy often means navigating a landscape of pain and discomfort. While lifestyle modifications and therapies play a crucial role in managing these symptoms, medications can be a valuable addition to your toolkit. Remember, medications are just one piece of the puzzle, and it's essential to work closely with your doctor to find the right balance for your unique needs.

Medications can be a lifeline for many people living with peripheral neuropathy, providing much-needed relief from pain and discomfort. They work by targeting different pain pathways and mechanisms within the body. Let's explore some common medications used for peripheral neuropathy pain relief:

Anticonvulsants: Initially developed to treat seizures, anticonvulsants like gabapentin and pregabalin have shown remarkable effectiveness in reducing nerve pain. They calm overactive nerves, diminishing the intensity and frequency of pain signals.

Antidepressants: While primarily used to treat depression, certain antidepressants, such as tricyclic antidepressants (TCAs) and serotonin-norepinephrine reuptake inhibitors (SNRIs), can also alleviate nerve pain. They work by modulating neurotransmitters in the brain, influencing pain perception.

Topical Medications: Creams, gels, or patches containing lidocaine or capsaicin can provide localized pain relief. Lidocaine numbs the area, while capsaicin desensitizes nerves over time, reducing pain signals.

Opioids: In some cases, stronger pain relievers like opioids might be considered for severe pain that doesn't respond to other treatments. However, due to their potential for dependence and side effects, they are typically reserved as a last resort and used cautiously.

While medications can offer significant relief, it's important to be aware of potential side effects. These can vary depending on the medication and individual responses. Common side effects include drowsiness, dizziness, dry mouth, constipation, and nausea. It's crucial to communicate openly with your doctor about any side effects you experience so that adjustments can be made if needed.

Remember, finding the right medication and dosage is a personalized journey. What works for one person may not work for another. Your doctor will consider various factors, including your medical history, other medications you're taking, and the severity of your pain, to tailor a treatment plan that's best for you.

It's important to note that medications are not a magic bullet, and they may not completely eliminate pain. However, they can significantly improve your quality of life by reducing pain intensity and allowing you to engage more fully in activities you enjoy.

As with any treatment, consistency is key. Take your medications as prescribed by your doctor, even if you start feeling better. Skipping doses or stopping abruptly can lead to a resurgence of pain or withdrawal symptoms.

If you're considering medication for your peripheral neuropathy pain, have an open and honest conversation with your doctor. Discuss the pros and cons of different options, potential side effects, and any concerns you may have. Together, you can create a pain management plan that empowers you to live a fulfilling life despite the challenges of peripheral neuropathy.

Remember, managing pain is an ongoing process. It may require adjustments along the way, but with the right support and a proactive approach, you can regain control and thrive with peripheral neuropathy. Don't hesitate to reach out to your healthcare team for guidance and support on this journey. They are there to help you navigate the complexities of pain management and find solutions that work best for you.

In our journey towards thriving with peripheral neuropathy, we've explored the power of lifestyle changes and medications. Now, let's delve into a realm of therapies that offer relief without the need for pills: non-pharmacological approaches. This trio of techniques—TENS, acupuncture, and physical therapy—can play a significant role in managing pain and enhancing your overall quality of life.

TENS: Your Personal Pain Zapper

Imagine having a mini pain-relief device at your fingertips. That's the magic of Transcutaneous Electrical Nerve Stimulation, or TENS for short. This portable device delivers gentle electrical impulses through electrodes placed on your skin. It might sound a bit sci-fi, but the science behind it is surprisingly simple. Those impulses work in two ways: they block pain signals traveling to your brain, and they stimulate your body to release endorphins, your natural painkillers.

TENS is like having your very own pain-zapping remote control. You can adjust the intensity and frequency of the impulses to find what feels best for you. Some people describe the sensation as a tingling or buzzing, while others find it more like a gentle massage. The beauty of TENS is that it's non-invasive and generally safe, making it a great option for many people with peripheral neuropathy.

Acupuncture: Ancient Wisdom for Modern Relief

Acupuncture, a cornerstone of traditional Chinese medicine, involves the insertion of thin needles at specific points on your body. While the thought of needles might seem intimidating, the sensation is usually quite mild. Many people even find it relaxing.

But how does sticking needles into your skin help with pain? Acupuncture is thought to work by stimulating nerves and triggering the release of endorphins. It's like a wake-up call for your body's own pain-relief system. Research suggests that acupuncture can be effective in reducing neuropathic pain, improving sleep, and enhancing overall well-being.

Physical Therapy: Your Path to Stronger Nerves

When you're living with peripheral neuropathy, it's easy to fall into a pattern of inactivity. But moving your body is crucial for nerve health. That's where physical therapy comes in. A physical therapist can design a personalized exercise program that helps improve strength, flexibility, balance, and coordination.

These exercises might not seem directly related to pain relief, but they work wonders by improving blood flow to your nerves, reducing inflammation, and strengthening the muscles that support your feet and legs. Think of it as giving your nerves a helping hand to heal and function better.

Beyond exercises, physical therapists can also teach you techniques for managing pain, such as desensitization therapy and gait training (how to walk more comfortably and safely). Physical therapy empowers you to take an active role in your recovery and reclaim your independence.

Finding Your Non-Pharmacological Dream Team

Remember, managing peripheral neuropathy is often a multi-pronged approach. Combining TENS, acupuncture, and physical therapy with lifestyle changes and medications can create a powerful synergy for pain relief and improved nerve function. Talk to your doctor about which of these therapies might be right for you. It's also important to seek out qualified practitioners who have experience working with people with diabetes and peripheral neuropathy.

Don't be afraid to experiment and find what works best for you. Each person's journey with peripheral neuropathy is unique, and your treatment plan should reflect that. Keep an open mind, explore your options, and don't underestimate the power of these non-pharmacological approaches. With the right tools and support, you can thrive despite your diagnosis and live a full, active life.

Real-Life Inspiration: John's Story

John, a 65-year-old retiree with type 2 diabetes, was struggling with the pain and numbness of peripheral neuropathy. He was hesitant to try medications due to their side effects. After consulting with his doctor, he decided to give TENS and physical therapy a try.

Within a few weeks, John noticed a significant reduction in his pain levels. He was able to walk longer distances without discomfort, and he even started gardening again, a hobby he had given up due to his neuropathy. The TENS unit became his trusty companion, providing relief whenever he needed it.

Inspired by his progress, John added acupuncture to his routine. He found that the combination of therapies not only helped with his pain but also improved his sleep and overall mood. John's story is a testament to the power of non-pharmacological approaches. It's a reminder that even without medications, there are effective ways to manage peripheral neuropathy and reclaim your life.

Style changes: how to get less pain and more joy

You may have heard that making changes to your lifestyle is very important if you have diabetic peripheral neuropathy. The things you eat, how much you move, and how stressed you are can all make a big difference in how you feel every day. This way of living is like making small adjustments to an instrument that is carefully tuned. These changes will help the instrument play its best tune.

Taking care of your nerves: the diabetic neuropathy diet

The food you eat does more than just fuel your body. It also gives your nerves the nutrients they need to stay healthy. A healthy, well-balanced diet can help you control your blood sugar, which is very important for keeping nerve damage from getting worse. Let's break it down into tasty steps that we can take.

• Eat lots of fruits and vegetables. They are full of antioxidants that help keep your brain healthy. You should try to eat a lot of different colored foods, like bright vegetables like peppers and carrots, nuts, and leafy greens.

• Pick whole grains: Instead of white bread, rice, and pasta, choose whole-grain versions. They have more fiber, which helps keep your blood sugar in check and makes you feel full.

• Protein Power: Fish, chicken, beans, and lentils are all lean protein sources that give your nerves the building blocks they need to heal.

• Healthy Fats: Don't stay away from fats, but be smart about what you eat. Pick nuts, seeds, bananas, and olive oil. They help your heart and brain.

• Eat less sugar and processed foods. These can raise your blood sugar and hurt your nerves. Carefully read labels and stay away from processed foods and foods with extra sugars.

Remember that this isn't about going without; it's about choosing foods that taste good, are good for you, and make you feel good. Try different tastes and new recipes until you find the ones that work best for you. A registered dietitian can help you make a meal plan that is unique to your wants and tastes.

On the Way to Relief: Exercise and Neuropathy

When you're in pain and discomfort, exercise might not seem like the best thing to do, but it can help you control your neuropathy. As a result of regular exercise, your blood flow can be improved, which brings oxygen and nutrients to your nerves and can help lessen pain and improve nerve function.

• Keep your blood sugar in check: working out makes your body use insulin better, which is very important for controlling diabetes.

• Improve your mood: When you work out, your body creates endorphins, which are chemicals that make you feel good and can help you relax.

• Get stronger: This can help you keep your balance and lower your risk of falling.

The important thing is to do things you enjoy that are also good for your health level. Start out slowly and slowly add more exercise as you get stronger. People with neuropathy can do a lot of great things, like walking, swimming, biking, and yoga. Talk to your doctor or a physical trainer if you don't know where to begin. They can help you make an exercise plan that is safe and works for you.

Live More, Stress Less: How to Deal with Stress for   Neuropathy

It can be stressful to have a long-term illness like neuropathy, and worry can make your symptoms worse. For your health's sake, you need to find healthy ways to deal with worry. Here are some ideas that could work:

Deep breathing, meditation, and progressive muscle relaxation are all relaxing techniques that can help calm your nervous system and lower your stress.

• Mindfulness: Being aware of the present moment can help you let go of stress and problems.

• Yoga and Tai Chi: These gentle exercises mix movement with mindful awareness and deep breathing, which helps you relax and feel less stressed.

• Joining a support group with people who understand what you're going through can be very helpful and energizing.

• Therapy: Talking to a therapist can help you learn how to deal with stress and build coping skills.

Don't forget that dealing with stress is a personal process. Some people may not be able to use something that works for someone else.

Try out different methods until you find the one that makes you feel calm and balanced. Plus, remember to be kind to yourself and know that dealing with a long-term illness takes time.

Your Way of Life, Your Choices

It's not always easy to change the way you live, but it's worth it. You can take charge of your neuropathy and make your life better by eating well, working out regularly, and learning how to deal with stress in a healthy way. Keep in mind that it's not about being great, but about getting better. Your happiness and health will improve with each good choice you make.

Always keep in mind that you're not the only one making changes to your life. Your family, friends, and healthcare team are all there to help you. When you need help, don't be afraid to ask for it. You can do well with peripheral neuropathy if you work together.

Chapter 3: Protecting Your Feet: A Step-by-Step Guide

The Importance of Daily Foot Inspections
You could think of your feet as the unsung stars of your body that get you through life. People with diabetes and peripheral neuropathy, on the other hand, need a little extra care and attention from these leaders. That's why daily foot checks are so important. They are easy but very effective.

At this point, you may be thinking, "What's all the fuss about daily checks?" Shouldn't I just check my feet every once in a while?" The reason is in the small changes that can happen because of peripheral neuropathy. You might not notice small cuts, blisters, or pressure points on your feet until they get worse because your feet don't feel as well.

Doing regular foot checks is like having an early notice system that lets you find these problems before they become big problems. What this means is that you're taking responsibility for your feet and can do things to keep them healthy. Remember that early detection is the key to avoiding problems and living a full, busy life.

Your daily routine for checking your feet

The foot inspection process can be broken down into a few easy steps:

1. Get your tools together: Place yourself in a well-lit room and make yourself comfortable. You can lie on your bed or sit in a chair. If you need to, get a mirror to see the bottoms of your feet clearly. For a better look, you can also use a magnifying glass.

2. Look for Changes: First, look at your feet to see if they have any cuts, sores, blisters, redness, swelling, or changes in the color or warmth of the skin. The space between your toes is prone to getting wet, so pay extra attention to that area.

3. Take a Stand for Diversity: Run your fingers slowly over the tops and bottoms of your feet with your hands. Check to see if there are any lumps, bumps, or changes in the material. Don't forget to look at your toes for signs of fungal infections or nails that have grown back into themselves.

4. Don't forget your shoes and socks. Check them for any foreign items, rough seams, or general wear and tear that could make your feet hurt. For your foot health, remember that shoes that fit well and are comfortable are essential.

Making it a Habit

Foot checks work best when they are done the same way every time. It should be something you do every day, like after you shower or before bed. To stay on track, you can even set an alarm on your phone or calendar. Self-care means taking a moment to connect with your body and make sure it's healthy.

Don't be afraid to call your healthcare provider if you notice anything out of the ordinary during your check. They can look at the situation and suggest the best way to treat or stop the problem. When it comes to your feet, remember that it's better to be safe than sorry.

After inspections, here are some more tips to keep your feet happy.

Daily checks of the feet are only one part of the problem. To keep your feet healthy and happy, here are some more tips:

• Every day, wash your feet: Warm water and light soap should be used. Make sure they are completely dry, especially between the toes.

• Put lotion on your feet: Use a light lotion to keep your skin from getting dry and cracking. Do not put oil in the space between your toes.

• Put on shoes that feel good: Pick shoes that fit well and give your feet enough support. Stay away from shoes that are too tight or have high heels.

• Keep your toes short: To avoid getting ingrown toenails, cut them straight across.

• Keep your feet safe from extremely hot or cold surfaces. Wear socks when it's cold outside and don't walk barefoot on hot surfaces.

By doing these things every day, you'll be doing a lot to protect your feet and live a more comfortable, busy life.

Your feet, the base of your body

Don't forget that your feet are what hold you up. They help you every step of the way as you go through life. By giving them the care and attention they need, you're not only protecting your health, but also putting money into your good health in general. And so, every day, take a moment to enjoy these amazing engineering feats and believe in the power of daily foot inspections. It will be good for your feet.

Footwear and nail care that are right are the building blocks of healthy feet.

People who have peripheral neuropathy don't have to give up the easy things they enjoy, like going for a walk in the park or going out to dance at night. It just means giving a little more attention to the little things, especially when it comes to your feet, which are the base of your mobility. We'll talk about how taking care of your feet and nails properly can change your daily life, making it more comfortable, avoiding problems, and even giving you a spring in your step.

Why Shoes Are Important: Not Just for Style

Think of your shoes as a shield that keeps your feet safe.

Getting the right pair can protect you from accidents, make your steps more comfortable, and even out the pressure. This defense is even more important for people with peripheral neuropathy. Because you may not feel as well in your feet, you might not notice a blister or small cut until it gets worse.

This is why shoes that fit well are important. They should be snug enough to keep your foot from moving around but not so tight that your toes can't move. So that moisture doesn't build up and cause fungal diseases, the material should be able to breathe. To ease the stress on your nerves and joints, choose shoes with good back support. Don't forget that the most expensive shoe might not be the best one for you.

Comfort and usefulness should come before dress   trends.
Your Shopping List for Shoes:

• Size: Because your foot size can change over time, you should always have a professional measure your feet. When your feet are a little swelled at the end of the day, try on shoes.

• Material: To keep moisture from building up, choose materials that let air pass through them, like leather or mesh.

• Fit: Leave enough space between your toes for them to move. So your foot doesn't slip out, the heel should fit tightly.

If you want to keep your feet from hurting, look for shoes with good arch support and padding.

• Style: Choose shoes with ends that you can change, like laces or Velcro straps, so you can make them fit just right.

• Specialty Footwear: If you have problems with your feet, like hammertoes or bunions, you might want to think about getting special orthotics or therapeutic shoes.

Remember that it may take some tries before you find the right shoes. Don't be afraid to get help from a podiatrist or shoe expert. They can help you find the best shoes for your feet.

Take Small Steps to Take Care of Your Nails

Nail care is an important part of foot health that is often forgotten. Because peripheral neuropathy makes it harder to feel and heal, even a small nail problem can get worse very quickly. This is why having your nails clean and trimmed can help a lot in avoiding problems.

How to Take Care of Your Nails:

• Trimming: Don't round the ends of your toenails; cut them straight across. This keeps your toenails from getting ingrown, which is painful when the nail grows into the skin.

• File: Use a nail file to smooth out any rough spots. How to Clean: Use warm water and soap to wash your feet every day. Make sure they are completely dry, especially between the toes.

• Moisturize: Put a soothing cream on your feet, but don't put it between your toes.

• Inspect: Look at your feet and nails often for cuts, sores, or changes in color. Talk to your doctor if you notice anything that doesn't seem right.

Remember that you should never be afraid to ask for help if you can't see or reach your feet. Someone you care about or a medical worker can help you with your nail care routine.

What Prevention Can Do for You

Taking care of your feet is good for your health in general. It has to do with avoiding problems, easing pain, and keeping your freedom. Remember that little steps can add up to big changes. You're not only protecting your feet when you take care of your nails and shoes every day; you're also giving yourself the tools you need to live a full and busy life with peripheral neuropathy. So, put on those shoes that feel good, take some time to care for your feet, and go out with confidence. It will be good for your feet.

How to Keep Your Feet Healthy and Avoid and Treat Foot Ulcers

People with diabetes often worry about getting foot sores, especially those who have peripheral neuropathy. They can be very troublesome, but they don't have to happen. You can take big steps to stop them and even heal ones that are already there with proactive care and some knowledge. This is your plan for keeping your feet healthy and lowering your risk of getting ulcers.

Understanding Foot Ulcers: Why Early Detection Is Key

Scars or spots on the feet often turn into ulcers over time. Neuropathy makes it hard to feel things, so these wounds might not be seen, which lets them get deeper and infected. That's why it's important to do regular foot checks. Check to see if the skin is broken, red, swollen, or really warm. Always remember that early discovery is key! The easier it is to fix a problem, the faster you notice it.

The best defense is to avoid getting hurt: Step-by-Step Foot Care Plan

Take care of your feet every day as a loving routine and a way to say thank you for all the amazing things they do. Just follow this easy plan:

1. Cleanse: Use lukewarm water and light soap to wash your feet every day. Don't scrub too hard, and be kind.

2. Moisturize: Use a good lotion to keep your skin soft and free of cracks, but don't put it between your toes.

3. Check: Look at your feet carefully, making sure to look at the tops, bottoms, sides, and spaces between your toes. If you need to see things that are hard to get to, use a mirror.

4. Protect yourself: Wear clean, dry socks made of a material that lets air pass through, like wool or cotton. Tight socks can cut off blood flow, so stay away from them.

5. Make smart choices about shoes: Choose shoes that fit well, are comfy, and have plenty of room for your toes. Stay away from shoes with open toes and high heels.

A Whole-Body Approach to Treating Foot Ulcers

Don't worry if you do get a foot sore. Please remember that most ulcers can heal with quick and proper care.

What you need to do is:

1. Talk to your doctor: You should get medical help right away. Your doctor will look at how bad the ulcer is and tell you what the best treatment is.

2. Take pressure off: It's important for healing that you don't put too much pressure on the hurt area. Your doctor may tell you to wear special shoes, supports, or even a wheelchair or crutches for a short time.

3. Clean the wound: Make sure the ulcer stays dry and clean. Your doctor will tell you the right way to clean and bandage the wound.

4. Take care of your blood sugar: It's important to keep your blood sugar levels in a healthy range so that you can heal and avoid getting sick.

5. Think about other treatments: Your doctor may suggest other treatments, such as medicines, wound dressings, or even hyperbaric oxygen therapy, depending on how bad the ulcer is.

Adopt a healthy way of life: Taking Care of Your Feet and Body

A healthy lifestyle is important for avoiding foot ulcers and improving overall health, in addition to taking care of your feet every day and getting treatment right away. Here are some important things to keep in mind:

• Take care of your diabetes: To keep your blood sugar levels in check, do what your doctor tells you about your food, exercise, and medicine.

• Give up smoking: Because it hurts circulation and takes longer to heal, smoking makes getting foot sores much more likely.

• Stay at a healthy weight. Being overweight puts extra stress on your feet, which raises the risk of getting   ulcers.

• Work out regularly: Being active on a regular basis is good for your health and blood flow, which includes your feet.

• Stay hydrated: To keep your face healthy and hydrated, drink a lot of water.

• Get your feet checked regularly. Getting your feet checked regularly by your doctor or therapist is especially important if you have neuropathy.

Today is the start of your path to healthier feet. Don't forget that you can take care of your feet and live a full, busy life. You can avoid getting foot ulcers and treat them well if they do happen by giving your feet proper care, living a healthy life, and seeing a doctor right away if you need to. Give your feet the care and attention they deserve because they carry you through life.

Chapter 4: Navigating Daily Challenges: Maintaining Independence

Adaptive Tools and Techniques for Daily Activities

You don't have to give up your freedom or the things you love to do because you have peripheral neuropathy. In fact, you can continue to do well even though you have this problem if you are creative and have the right tools. Think of it as a new adventure where you have to change and find new ways to do things. This part is like a treasure map; it's full of useful tips that will help you get through your daily tasks with confidence and ease.

Easy Ways to Dress

We all know how good it feels to put together the right outfit, but for people with peripheral neuropathy, getting dressed can be a pain. The good news is that there are many tools that can make getting dressed very easy.

Reachers and grabbers can make things a lot easier. They make it easy to pull up your socks or pants or even reach things on high shelves. With button hooks and zipper pulls, it's easy to close clothes, and shoe horns with long handles take away the need to bend over.

Try out different styles of clothes. Most of the time, Velcro and elastic waistbands are easier to use than buttons and zippers. Shoes with wide openings and closures that can be adjusted can save your life. So can types that you can slip on. Also, don't forget about adaptive clothing brands that make designs that are comfy and easy to wear.

Adventures in cooking

A lot of people enjoy cooking, and neuropathy shouldn't get in the way of that. If you have trouble holding utensils, look for ones with built-in handles or ones made for people with arthritis. One rocking action is all it takes to use a rocker knife, and cutting boards with spikes that hold food in place and non-slip bases can help keep you from cutting yourself. A lot of cooking tools are also available to make preparing food easier. You might find jar openers, electric can openers, and automatic stirrers useful in your kitchen.

Bathing Bliss

Taking care of your health is very important, and there are many tools that can make bathing safer and more fun. Putting up grab bars near the toilet and in the shower can help people feel more stable. Shower chairs and benches let you sit easily while you bathe, which makes it less likely that you will trip and fall. You can reach your back and feet better with sponges and brushes that have long handles. Soap makers

with pump tops are also easier to use than regular soap bars.
If you want to avoid slipping and falling, use a non-slip bathmat. If it's hard for you to get in and out of the tub, a transfer bench can help.

Keeping moving

Keeping your mobility is important for your freedom, and there are lots of tools that can help you. Canes, walkers, and rollators can help with balance and support. Wheelchairs are better for longer routes or when walking is hard.

A stairlift can make your life so much easier if you have trouble going up and down stairs. To make your home easier to get into, you can also put in ramps. Accept technology. In this digital era, technology provides many useful tools for daily use. Voice-activated helpers can help you manage your smart home's lights, thermostats, and other devices.

Medication reminder apps can make sure you never miss a dose. Voice-to-text software and apps that magnify text can make reading and writing easier. You might want to look into support groups and boards online. Meeting people who understand what you're going through can give you a lot of strength and be a great source of information and support.

Do not forget that having peripheral neuropathy does not mean you have to stop doing the things you enjoy. It's about coming up with creative new ways to do them. Take on the task, look into the options, and keep doing well! You can stay independent and live a full life if you have the right tools and an upbeat attitude.

Things that work best for you are the ones you need to find. Try out different choices, and don't be afraid to ask your doctor, occupational therapist, or other health care worker for help. They can give you specific advice and help you find your way around adaptive tools.

Remember that you are not alone most of all. There is a lot of knowledge and help out there for the millions of people who live with peripheral neuropathy. Reach out to other people, make connections, and be positive and strong as you start a new part of your life.

Safe Ways to Move Around and Avoid Falling

You don't have to give up your freedom if you have peripheral neuropathy. You can easily and safely move through the world by making small changes to your daily routine and the places you visit. This part will give you useful tips on how to improve your mobility and lower your risk of falling. This will help you keep doing the things you love and living a full life.

How Your Body Works and Neuropathy

To move around safely, you must first understand how peripheral neuropathy impacts your body. Neuropathy can make it hard to feel your feet, keep your balance, and coordinate your moves because it causes numbness, tingling, and pain. This can cause people to trip or fall, especially in difficult places or when they need to be very precise. After learning about these problems, you can take steps to avoid accidents and keep your freedom.

Looking at your surroundings

First, pay more attention to what's around you. Are there any possible dangers in your home or job that could make you more likely to fall? Things like loose rugs, cluttered paths, uneven floors, or not enough light could be examples of this. You can get rid of or make these dangers safer by figuring out what they are. For instance, use double-sided tape to hold down loose rugs, clear walks of clutter, fix surfaces that aren't level, and add more light to areas that aren't getting enough.

Getting Your Home Ready

Simple changes to your home can make it much safer and easier for you to move around. You might want to put up grab bars in the bathroom, steps on the stairs, and non-slip mats in the bathtub or shower. You could also move furniture around to make paths bigger, get rid of walls that separate rooms, and use nightlights to make things easier to see at night. By making changes to your home, you make it better, which helps you stay independent and lowers your risk of falling.

How to Pick the Right Shoes

Getting the right shoes can help you stay stable and balanced. Choose shoes that don't slip, have good hip support, and fit well. If you don't want to trip or fall, don't wear high heels, flip-flops, or shoes with backs that are loose or open. If you want to feel good, pick shoes with a wide, stable base and a low heel. You might want to talk to a doctor or someone who specializes in shoes to get advice on the shoes that will work best for you.

Keeping your strength and balance

You're less likely to fall if you work out regularly because it makes your muscles stronger, your balance better, and your agility better. You might want to add things like walking, swimming, yoga, or tai chi to your schedule. These exercises can help you get in better shape generally, improve your balance, and make your leg muscles stronger. Stand on one leg or walk from heel to toe are two easy workouts that can help. Before you start a new workout plan, you should talk to your doctor.

Using Devices to Help

If you have a hard time keeping your balance or moving around, assistance devices like canes, walkers, or crutches can help you stay stable and supported. These things can help you keep your balance, make walking easier on your legs, and boost your confidence. It's important to learn how to use your aid device correctly and pick the right one for your needs. A physical therapist can help you choose the right assistive equipment and make sure it works well for you.

Keeping busy and active

For your physical and mental health, it's important to keep a busy lifestyle. Do not let peripheral neuropathy stop you from doing things. Keep doing the things you love doing for fun and for social reasons. This can help you feel better, be less stressed, and keep your freedom. If neuropathy means you have to change the things you do, get creative and find other ways to stay busy. For instance, if you like hiking, think about going on shorter trails that aren't as hard, or walk with a group for support.

How to Deal with Pain and Illness

Peripheral neuropathy can cause pain and discomfort that can make it hard to move around and raise your risk of falling. Taking good care of your symptoms is important if you want to keep your freedom and quality of life. This could mean taking prescription drugs, over-the-counter pain killers, heat or cold therapy, or trying unusual treatments like massage or acupuncture. Talk to your doctor about how to deal with your pain in a way that works for you.

Check-ups every month

You need to see your doctor regularly to keep an eye on your neuropathy and deal with any problems that come up. Your doctor can check how mobile you are, suggest the right treatments, and help you come up with ways to keep from falling. Tell your doctor about any changes in your symptoms or worries you have about being able to move around.

These tips will help you deal with the problems that come with peripheral neuropathy and keep your freedom. Don't forget that you have friends and family. You can keep living a full and busy life if you have the right tools, support, and attitude.

Making changes to your home to make it safer

Being independent and safe at home don't have to be hard to deal with if you have peripheral neuropathy. By making a few thoughtful changes, you can make your home safe and comfortable in a way that meets your specific needs and helps you grow. This section will talk about useful changes you can make to your home to make it safer, lower your risk of falling, and make your life better in general. Remember that a few changes made in the right places can make a huge difference.

Making the bathroom safer

Bathrooms can be hard for people with peripheral neuropathy because of the hard surfaces and the chance of getting wet. Luckily, making a few easy changes can make things a lot safer. Put grab bars near the toilet and in the shower or bathtub to start. These strong rails give support and steadiness, which lowers the risk of falling. You might want to put non-slip mats or adhesive strips on the floor of the shower or bathroom to make it safer and easier to walk on.

If it's hard for you to step over the edge of a regular bathtub, you might want to get a walk-in tub or shower instead. You don't have to step over a high threshold to use these accessible choices. This makes bathing safer and easier. You might also want to put in a higher toilet seat, which will make it easier to sit down and stand up.

Making the kitchen safer

The kitchen is a place where lots of people gather to eat and do things. It can also be changed to make it safer and easier for people with peripheral neuropathy to use. Start by setting up your kitchen so that everything is easy to get to. Put things you use often close at hand so you don't have to bend over or climb to get to them. For jobs that need you to stand, choose sturdy stools or chairs with backrests to make sure you have the right support and stability.

You could put pull-out shelves or drawers in lower cabinets to make it easier to get to things without having to bend over or reach deep inside. Lever-style handles are easier to hold and move around than standard knobs and faucets. You might also want to buy kitchen tools that are made to help people who have trouble moving their fingers, like jar openers, rocker knives, and tools with built-in handles.

Changing the way you live

You might want to make a few key changes to your home to make it safer and easier to get to. First, get rid of any clutter and make sure the paths are clear and unblocked. Tighten up any rugs or mats that aren't attached to the floor to keep people from tripping. You might want to put nightlights in the halls and bathrooms to help you find your way at night.

In case your home has steps, make sure they are well-lit and have strong handrails. If going up and down stairs gets hard, you might want to install a step lift or look into other ways to live on one level. If you use a wheelchair or walker, you might want to add ramps or widen doorways to make your home easier to get around in.

Looking for Professional Help

You can make many changes to your home on your own, but it's usually best to talk to a professional, like an occupational therapist or a builder who specializes in making homes more accessible. These professionals can look at your unique needs, make suggestions based on those needs, and walk you through the steps of making your home safer and more useful.

Remember that making changes to your home is an investment in your health, safety, and freedom. By being aware of possible dangers and putting practical solutions in place, you can make your living space one that helps you grow while dealing with the challenges of peripheral neuropathy.

Extra Tips to Make Things Safer

Besides making changes to the structure, there are other things you can do to make your house safer:

• Look over your shoes often: Make sure your shoes are in good shape, have soles that won't slip, and fit right.
• Make sure there is enough light: Having enough lights in your home is very important for safety. If you can't see well in some places, you might want to add more lamps or brighter lights.

Keep things in order: Keeping your living areas clean and free of clutter will make it less likely that you will trip or fall over things that you have lost.

• Make regular exercise a priority. Regular exercise can improve your balance, coordination, and general strength, which lowers your risk of falling.

• Let your loved ones know: Tell your family and friends about your worries and limits so they know what you need and can help you when you need it.

You don't have to give up safety or freedom to live with peripheral neuropathy. You can make your home a safe and supportive place to live that helps you grow by making changes ahead of time and using practical strategies.

Don't forget that your home should be a safe place where you can unwind, recover, and fully enjoy life. Making changes to your home is an investment in your health and an openness to a future full of opportunities.

Chapter 5: The Diabetes-Neuropathy Connection: Understanding the Risks

How High Blood Sugar Damages Nerves
Neuropathy is the medical term for nerve damage. If you have had diabetes for a while, you may have heard that it may be linked to sugar. Although the thought of this problem may be scary, knowing how it happens can give you the power to take charge of your health and lower your risk of nerve damage.

How does having high blood sugar hurt nerves, then?

Think of your nerves as a complex system of roads that carry important information all over your body. Like a traffic jam that won't go away, high blood sugar gets in the way of this smooth flow of conversation. Over time, this constant interference can hurt the delicate nerve cells, which can cause different neuropathy symptoms.
One of the main ways that high blood sugar hurts your nerves is by making them swell up. Inflammation is like your body's alarm system; it goes off when it gets hurt or irritated. Inflammation is an important part of keeping your body safe, but long-term inflammation from having regularly high blood sugar can hurt nerves and make them less effective.

Another way that high blood sugar hurts nerves is by taking away nutrients that are necessary for nerve health. These nutrients, along with vitamins and minerals, get to your brain through your bloodstream. Having high blood sugar, on the other hand, can stop this process, leaving your nerves without food. High blood sugar can hurt the tiny blood vessels that bring oxygen and nutrients to your nerves, as well as cause inflammation and nutrient loss. These tiny blood tubes, which are called capillaries, keep your nerves alive. When high blood sugar hurts these vessels, it limits the flow of oxygen and nutrients to your nerves, which makes nerve damage worse.

Now, let's look at the exact ways that nerve damage is caused by high blood sugar. An important part of this process is a chemical known as sorbitol. If you have too much glucose (sugar) in your blood, some of it is changed into sorbitol in your nerve cells. Sorbitol can build up inside cells, which makes them swell by drawing in water. This swelling can hurt the nerve fibers and make it harder for them to send messages correctly.

Additionally, having high blood sugar can cause certain enzymes in your nerve cells to work, which create dangerous substances known as free radicals. Free radicals are molecules that respond very quickly and can hurt the structure and function of cells. This reactive stress, which is brought on by too many free radicals, can make nerve damage worse.

The creation of advanced glycation end products (AGEs) is another thing that can lead to nerve damage. AGEs are made when too many sugar molecules link to proteins in your body, like those in nerve cells. AGEs can cross-link with proteins, which makes them stiff and unable to do their job. This process can stop nerve cells from working normally and make nerve damage worse. There are different ways that high blood sugar can hurt brain health. You could feel tingling or stiffness in your feet or hands, as well as sharp pains or weak muscles. Nerve damage can sometimes affect your internal systems, causing problems with your digestive system, urinary tract, or heart.

The bad things that could happen if you hurt your nerves might be too much to handle, but you can change how healthy your nerves are. You can greatly lower your chance of getting neuropathy and keep your nerves from getting worse by keeping an eye on your blood sugar levels and living a healthy life.

A balanced diet and routine exercise are two of the best ways to keep your blood sugar levels in check. Limit the amount of processed foods, sugary drinks, and unhealthy fats you eat and make sure your meals are full of fruits, veggies, and whole grains. A lot of regular exercise, like brisk walking, swimming, or riding, can make your body more sensitive to insulin, a hormone that helps control blood sugar.

Besides what you eat and how much you move, some medicines can also help you control your blood sugar and lower your risk of nerve damage. Based on your wants and health history, your doctor can help you figure out the best way to take your medications. Also, you should see your doctor regularly and keep an eye on your blood sugar levels on a regular basis. If you stay on top of managing your diabetes, you can spot any early signs of nerve damage and move quickly to stop more problems.

It may seem hard to live with diabetes and the risk of neuropathy, but know that you're not the only one. Millions of people around the world are going through the same thing, and there are a lot of tools and support networks out there to help you do well. You can give yourself the power to live a full and healthy life with diabetes by putting your health first, getting help from medical professionals, and making connections with people who understand what you're going   through.
Don't forget that information is power. You can protect your nerve health and keep enjoying all that life has to offer if you know how high blood sugar hurts nerves and take steps to control your diabetes.

How Important It Is to Control Blood Sugar

Keeping your blood sugar levels in a healthy range is like taking care of a precious garden. You have to pay attention, be dedicated, and really understand what's going on. This kind of careful nurturing is even more important for people who have diabetes and peripheral neuropathy. We'll look at the important connection between controlling your blood sugar and neuropathy in this chapter and explain why it's so important for people with this disease to do so. Your nerves are like a network of complicated paths that send messages all over your body. If your blood sugar stays high for a long time, it's like a storm is building over these nerve paths, damaging them and causing tingling, numbness, pain, and other neuropathy symptoms. There is good news, though:

You can change the way the weather works.

Figuring out the science behind the link

Researchers have found a strong link between having high blood sugar and getting peripheral neuropathy and making it worse. Hyperglycemia, or high blood sugar, sets off a chain of events in the body that can hurt nerve cells. Advanced glycation end products (AGEs) and oxidative stress are two examples of this.

AGEs and oxidative stress both cause nerve damage. Think of your nerves as thin wires. Over time, these wires get frayed and less good at sending signals when they are exposed to high amounts of sugar. This can cause the problems with feeling and pain that are typical of neuropathy. But if you take good care of your blood sugar, you're basically keeping these wires from getting worse and giving them a chance to heal.

What Prevention Can Do for You

Keeping blood sugar under control is very important if you want to avoid or delay the development of peripheral neuropathy. Studies have shown that people whose blood sugar levels are well controlled are less likely to get neuropathy than people whose levels are not well controlled. In other words, if you keep your blood sugar in a healthy range, you greatly lower your chance of feeling the painful symptoms that come with this condition.

Picture yourself starting a trip. Keeping your blood sugar levels at a healthy level is like picking a path with fewer bumps. You are giving yourself the best chance of avoiding the problems that come with neuropathy and living a more comfortable, busy life.

Getting in Charge of Your Health

Controlling your blood sugar is more than just reading a meter. It's about giving yourself the tools you need to take charge of your health. Making choices that are good for your health and help you do well even though you have diabetes and neuropathy is important. This needs a multifaceted method that includes:

• Eating well: A balanced diet full of fruits, veggies, whole grains, and lean protein can help keep your blood sugar levels steady and give your body the nutrients it needs to heal and grow.

• Going to the gym regularly: Being active makes your body use insulin better, which drops blood sugar. Aim to work out at a reasonable level for at least 30 minutes most days of the week.

• Sticking to your medications: If your doctor has given you diabetes medicine, it's very important that you take it exactly as told to keep your blood sugar under control.

• Checking Your Blood Sugar: If you check your blood sugar levels often, you can see how you're doing, find trends, and make changes as needed.

• Dealing with stress: Long-term stress can make blood sugar levels go up, so it's important to find good ways to deal with it, like yoga, meditation, or spending time in nature.

A Journey of Giving Power

Don't forget that you're not going through this trip by yourself. Your healthcare team is there to help you figure out how to control your blood sugar. They can help you achieve by giving you advice, support, and the right tools. You can make a personalized plan that fits your wants and goals if you work together.

Keeping your blood sugar levels in a healthy range is an ongoing process that has huge benefits. Controlling your blood sugar is important for your overall health and well-being as well as lowering your chance of neuropathy. You're looking forward to a life full of energy, strength, and the freedom to do what you love. Let's go on this journey together, with knowledge, determination, and the firm opinion that you can do well even though you have peripheral neuropathy.

Getting regular checkups and screenings: How to Take Charge of Your Success

Living a full life with peripheral neuropathy, especially when it's linked to diabetes, is a process of taking charge of your health and feeling empowered. See it like a beautiful hike where you can enjoy the scenery and know how to get around every turn with the best map and tools. These important tools are regular checkups and screenings, which give you useful information about your health and allow you to make smart decisions about your well-being.

Your health guide: the power of early detection Checkups should be thought of as a guide that points you in the direction of good health. They give you a chance to talk to your healthcare team about any changes or worries you may have and get advice that is specific to your needs. These checkups aren't just for keeping current conditions under control; they're also meant to stop problems from happening in the first place. Early detection is a key part of proactive health because it lets people get treatments and interventions at the right time, which can greatly improve results.

Foot Exams: Taking Care of Your Base

People with diabetes need to have their feet checked all the time. Most of the time, peripheral neuropathy starts in the feet. Getting your feet checked regularly can help find early signs of nerve damage, blood problems, or skin changes. You can take steps to protect your feet and avoid problems like sores or infections if you catch these problems early. Think of your feet as the basis of a house. They need to be cared for and maintained regularly to stay strong and stable.

A Holistic Approach to Comprehensive Diabetes Management

During your monthly checkups, they do more than just look at your neuropathy. They are part of a full plan for managing your diabetes that looks at all of your health. This means keeping an eye on your cholesterol, blood sugar, blood pressure, and other important signs. Imagine a symphony, where each instrument is very important to making the whole sound good. A holistic method to managing diabetes makes sure that you're not just taking care of your symptoms, but also getting to the root causes and improving your health as a whole.

Screening tests: Giving you a clear picture of your health

Along with checkups, screens are very important for getting a clear picture of your health. These tests can help find problems before they show up as symptoms. This lets you start treatment and control sooner. For instance, regular eye checks can find diabetic retinopathy, an eye problem, and kidney function tests can find out how healthy your kidneys are. By looking for and fixing possible problems before they happen, you're not only taking care of current health problems, but also protecting your health in the future.

Your healthcare team is there to help you stay healthy.
Don't forget that you're not going through this trip by yourself. Your healthcare team is committed to your health and will be there for you every step of the way. They can answer your questions, deal with your concerns, and give you advice that is specific to your wants. Don't be afraid to share your thoughts and experiences, ask questions, and be involved in the decisions that affect your health. By encouraging open conversation and teamwork, you're not only getting care, but also helping to make a way for everyone to thrive.

Taking Charge of Your Health: Giving You Power

Checkups and screenings should not just be seen as medical visits; they should also be seen as chances to gain power. When you take care of your health, you're not just dealing with conditions; you're also changing your well-being. Imagine that you are the captain of a ship that you are steering toward good health and endless opportunities. You're getting more useful information with each checkup and screening, which helps you make smart choices and plan a path to a happy life.

If you have peripheral neuropathy or diabetes, regular checkups and tests are the threads that hold together a picture of good health. By using these preventative tools, you're not just keeping things in order; you're thriving.

Don't forget that your health is the most important thing you have, and that spending money on it is like investing in your future. You're not just checking off boxes with each checkup and test; you're also taking steps toward a full and healthy life.

Chapter 6: Nutrition for Nerve Health: Fueling Your Body Right

The Role of Vitamins and Minerals
Have you ever thought about how the food you eat can hurt your nerves? It's not enough to just stay away from sugar and eat more vegetables. When you have diabetes or other health problems, the vitamins and minerals you eat can have a big effect on your feelings. This section will go into detail about vitamins and show you how important they are for nerve health. It will also help you choose a diet that will help you on your journey with peripheral neuropathy.

The first group is the B vitamins, which are also known as the "nerve vitamins." It is very important to get enough thiamine (B1), pyridoxine (B6), and cobalamin (B12). Thiamine is an important part of nerve communication and making energy, and pyridoxine helps make neurotransmitters, which are chemicals that send messages between nerve cells. Myelin is the protected covering around your nerves. You need cobalamin to make and keep it in good shape.

Your brain's myelin is like the coating around a wire. Electrical signals can't move well when this insulation is damaged or thin, which can cause numbness, tingling, or pain. Making sure you get enough B vitamins is like helping to keep the padding on your nerves in good shape.

So, where can you get these B vitamins that are good for nerves? Thankfully, they can be found in many foods. Eat a lot of whole grains, beans, nuts, and seeds to get thiamine. Chicken, fish, bananas, and potatoes all have a lot of pyridoxine. When it comes to cobalamin, you can mostly find it in meat, fish, eggs, and cheese. To get the B12 you need if you are a vegan or vegetarian, you might want to try fortified foods or pills.

When it comes to other important vitamins, vitamin E is the star. It's a strong antioxidant that keeps your cells safe from free radicals, which are dangerous molecules that can make your nerves go crazy. Vitamin E is like a shell that protects your nerves from the damage that oxidative stress can do.

Adding foods like nuts, seeds, spinach, and avocado to your diet can help you get more vitamin E. These not only give you vitamin E but also help you eat in a way that is good for your heart, which is important for controlling diabetes and keeping your nerves from getting worse.

Let's turn our attention to rocks now. For nerves to work well, magnesium, calcium, and potassium are especially important. A lot of nerve signals and muscle rest depend on magnesium. Calcium, on the other hand, helps nerves send signals and neurotransmitters get released. Potassium helps your nerve cells keep the right amount of electricity, which makes transmission go smoothly.

You can get a lot of magnesium from nuts, seeds, leafy green veggies, and whole grains. Plant-based milks that have been boosted with calcium and leafy greens can all help you get the calcium you need. Bananas, potatoes, spinach, and beans are all great foods that are high in potassium.

Remember that a healthy diet full of different fruits and veggies, whole grains, and lean proteins can give your nerves most of the vitamins and minerals they need. A trained dietitian or your doctor should help you figure out what to eat if you have diabetes or other dietary restrictions. They can look at your specific needs and, if necessary, suggest the right vitamins for you.

Getting these vitamins and minerals every day isn't just a way to control your peripheral neuropathy; it's also a way to live a healthier life that benefits your general health. Giving your nerves the tools they need to grow means taking care of your body from the inside   out.
Don't forget that you're not going through this trip by yourself. Millions of people have peripheral neuropathy. You can control your symptoms and live a full, happy life with the right information and help. So, believe in the power of food, give your body what it needs, and take action to live a better life with peripheral neuropathy.

How to Feed Your Nerves with Meal Planning and Healthy Recipes

It can be hard to find your way around when you have diabetes and peripheral neuropathy. Your food, on the other hand, is a strong weapon that can help you on this path. You can take care of your nerves, keep your blood sugar levels in check, and overall improve your quality of life by making smart food choices and planning your meals. This part will talk about planning meals and finding healthy recipes that are especially good for people with diabetes and peripheral neuropathy.

How to Understand the Power of Planning Your Meals

Planning your meals can help you find your way in the kitchen. It means planning your meals and snacks ahead of time to make sure they meet your health goals and nutritional needs. This method not only saves you time and money, but it also makes it less tempting to make bad decisions on the spot. You're more likely to make decisions that are good for your nerves and blood sugar when you have a plan.

Set aside some time once a week to come up with meal ideas. Think about what you like to eat, your cultural background, and any special needs you may have. At each meal, try to get a good blend of carbs, protein, and healthy fats. Eat a lot of fiber-rich foods, like fruits, veggies, whole grains, and legumes. They can help keep your blood sugar levels in check and improve your health in general.

Building a Base of Nutrient-Dense Ingredients

Let's look at the parts of a neuropathy-friendly diet now that you have a plan. Pay attention to foods that are high in nutrients and give you the vitamins, minerals, and antioxidants you need. It is very important for nerve health, repair, and defense that you get these nutrients. Leafy greens like spinach, kale, and collard greens are full of B vitamins, which your nerves need to work properly. You can put them in smoothies, salads, or meals that you sauté.

Berries like blueberries, strawberries, and raspberries have a lot of antioxidants that help fight oxidative stress, which can damage nerves. You can eat them as a snack, mix them into yogurt, or make a drink with them.

Omega-3 fatty acids can be found in large amounts in fatty fish like salmon, tuna, and mackerel. These acids can help reduce nerve pain and inflammation. You should try to eat them at least twice a week. Peanuts, walnuts, chia seeds, and flaxseeds are just a few of the nuts and seeds that are high in healthy fats, fiber, and vitamin E, which is known for being an antioxidant. For an extra healthy boost, sprinkle them on your yogurt, salads, or cereal.

Making recipes that are both tasty and good for you Now comes the fun part: making these healthy foods into meals that taste great and fill you up. The good news is that living healthy doesn't have to be dull or hard to do. You can make meals that are both tasty and good for you if you get creative and get ideas. Breakfast:

• Berry, nut, and seed oatmeal: An oatmeal bowl that makes you feel good is a great way to start the day. Put some of your favorite berries on top, along with some nuts and seeds and a drizzle of honey or maple syrup to make it taste sweet.

• Place Greek yogurt, granola, and fresh fruit in a glass one on top of the other. This is a quick and easy breakfast that is high in protein and fiber.

• Scrambled eggs with vegetables: Add your best vegetables, like peppers, mushrooms, and spinach, to eggs and mix them together. Top with cheese.

Lunch:

• Salad with chicken or fish that has been grilled. A salad is a cool and healthy lunch choice. It has a lot of fiber and nutrients from the greens. Add grilled chicken or fish on top for extra protein.

• Lentil soup with whole-wheat bread: Lentil soup is a rich, filling meal that is high in fiber and protein. For a full meal, serve it with a slice of whole-wheat bread.

• A bowl of quinoa with roasted veggies and hummus. Quinoa is a good source of fiber and all nine essential amino acids. For a tasty and full lunch, eat it with hummus and roasted vegetables.

Dinner: baked salmon with roasted veggies. Salmon is a healthy fish that tastes great and is easy to bake. For a full meal, serve it with roasted veggies like broccoli, carrots, and Brussels sprouts.

• Brown rice and chicken stir-fry: A stir-fry is a quick and easy way to make a healthy meal. For a healthy meal, mix lean chicken with your favorite veggies and brown rice.

• Chili is a hearty and warming meal that's great for a cold night. Try vegetarian chili with whole-wheat bread. • With a piece of whole-wheat bread, serve it as a vegetarian dish with beans, lentils, and salad.

These are only some thoughts to get you going. You can make a lot of other tasty and healthy meals with ingredients that are high in nutrients.

In conclusion:

Don't forget that your diet is a process, not a goal. It means making long-term decisions that are good for your body and your health as a whole. You can take charge of your health and do well with diabetes and peripheral neuropathy if you plan your meals, choose foods that are high in nutrients, and make tasty recipes.

Stay away from foods that make neuropathy worse. What you eat is like a secret tool that can help you fight peripheral neuropathy. It gives your body power and can also help your symptoms. However, did you know that some things can make neuropathy worse? These foods are like kryptonite; you need to stay away from them just like she does.

Your Enemy, Sugar: Having too much sugar in your blood can hurt your nerves and make your neuropathy symptoms worse. It's like adding more wood to the fire. Our blood sugar goes up when we eat sugary foods, which can hurt nerves over time. It's important to stay away from or limit prepared foods, cookies, candies, and drinks with a lot of sugar. Remember that fruits and veggies have natural sugars that are fine to eat in small amounts because they are also full of fiber and other nutrients. There is a hidden danger in refined grains: Refined carbs like white bread, rice, and pastries can make your blood sugar rise in the same way that sugary foods do. They've been stripped of their fiber and nutrients, leaving behind a food high in carbs that your body turns into sugar quickly. It can make a big difference to switch to whole carbs like brown rice, quinoa, and whole-wheat bread. Because these grains are digested slowly, they help keep your brain healthy and your blood sugar level steady.

Two strikes against fried and processed foods: A lot of the time, these foods have a lot of sugar, salt, and bad fats, all of which can make inflammation worse and neuropathy symptoms worse. They are like the bad guys in the world of food; they make you crazy. Think of fried foods as little gremlins that make your body swell up and cause nerve pain. On the other hand, processed foods often have a lot of salt, which can make you retain water and squash your nerves.

Alcohol, a Tricky Enemy: Most people can drink alcohol in moderation without getting sick, but people with neuropathy should avoid it. Alcohol can hurt nerves directly, making pain and other signs worse. Moderation is key if you like to drink once in a while.

Remember that drinking can make you thirstier, which can make nerve sensations worse.

This makes you wonder, "What's left to eat?" Don't worry—many tasty and healthy foods can help ease the effects of your neuropathy. Some of these are:

• Fruits and vegetables: these are full of minerals, vitamins, and antioxidants that are good for brain health. They are like the superheroes of food—they protect you from harm and keep your nerves healthy.

• Lean protein: Chicken, fish, and beans are all good sources of this protein. They give your body the building blocks it needs to repair nerves.

Healthy fats: These fats can lower inflammation and protect nerves. You can find them in foods like nuts, eggs, and olive oil.

At first, switching to a healthier diet might seem hard. But remember that it's a trip, not a race. Start slowly and make small changes to the way you eat. Try out new recipes, find new tastes, and find healthy foods that you like. Food that is good for you is an investment in your health.

To make the change easy, here are some tips:
• Pay close attention to food labels: Watch out for secret sugars, fats that are bad for you, and too much sodium.

• Cook at home more often. This way, you can choose the foods you use and how they are cooked.

• Make a list of your snacks and meals: This can help you stay away from making hasty, bad decisions.
• Don't be shy about asking for help: A registered dietitian can help you make a meal plan that is unique to your wants and tastes.

Don't forget that every healthy choice you make, no matter how small, helps your nerves. You can take charge of your neuropathy symptoms and live a fuller, more healthy life by staying away from foods that make them worse and eating healthier foods instead.

You are not only dealing with your neuropathy; you are living in spite of it. You are on this trip, and you can make it a success if you know what to do and have the right tools.

Chapter 7: Exercise for Neuropathy: Move Your Way to Better Health

Safe and Effective Exercise Options

It might seem hard to start working out when you have peripheral neuropathy, but remember that you won't become a marathon runner overnight. It's about getting stronger, having fun with moving, and making your health better in general. You will be amazed at how far you can go with a well-thought-out exercise plan that is made just for you. Let us look at some safe and successful ways for people with diabetes and peripheral neuropathy to work out.

Walking: The First Thing You Can Do to Get Healthy

There's a good reason why walking is often seen as the most important part of any workout plan. It's easy for almost everyone to do, doesn't hurt, and is great for your physical and mental health. Walking every day can help your heart health, make your muscles stronger, and improve your happiness. Start slowly, like with a 10-minute walk around your area. As you gain confidence, slowly increase the length and intensity of your workouts.

Dive into fitness with water aerobics

Water yoga might be the best way to work out if you want to do something easy on your joints. It's easier to move around and work out in water because it makes you float, which lessens the effect on your feet and legs. There are usually a lot of different movements in water aerobics classes that work out all of your muscles. Also, the social part of group classes can really help you stick with it.

Getting Balance and Harmony with Tai Chi and Yoga

Yoga and Tai Chi are both very old practices that involve slow, mindful moves and deep breathing. A lot of people with peripheral neuropathy need to work on their flexibility, balance, and coordination. These routines can help. Tai chi and yoga can both help you rest and feel less stressed, which is good for your health as a whole. A lot of gyms and community centers have lessons just for beginners, which makes it easy to start.

Strength training will make you stronger.

When you think of exercise for neuropathy, strength training might not be the first thing that comes to mind, but it's an important part of a well-rounded fitness plan. Getting stronger muscles can help you keep your balance, lower your risk of falling, and make your body work better in general. To avoid getting hurt, start with light weights or resistance bands and pay attention to your form. To make sure you're doing exercises safely and correctly, working

with a skilled trainer can be very helpful. You can pedal your way to better health with stationary cycling.
One more low-impact exercise that's easy on the joints is stationary riding. It's a great way to burn calories, strengthen your legs, and keep your heart healthy. You can find stationary bikes at a lot of gyms and exercise centers, or you can buy one to keep at home. Start with short, easy workouts and slowly add more time and effort as you get stronger.

When you dance, follow your heart's beat.

Work out can be fun, right? Dancing is a fun way to move your body and get your heart rate up. Dancing can help your heart health, coordination, and balance, whether you like ballroom dancing, salsa, or just moving to your favorite music at home. It's also a great way to relax and feel better.

Pay attention to your body.

Always remember that paying attention to your body is the most important part of any workout plan. If you feel any pain or soreness, change how active you are to account for it. Being nice to yourself and not pushing yourself too hard are important. Just remember that everyone has good and bad days. Talk to your doctor if you have any strange signs during or after exercise.

The Power of Being Stable

When it comes to getting the most out of exercise, consistency is key. Aim to work out at a reasonable level for at least 30 minutes most days of the week. It's possible to split it up into shorter lessons if that works better for you. Getting daily exercise is what matters.

Find what drives you.

It can be hard to get yourself to work out, but it's worth the effort. Think about what drives you. It could be that you want to feel better in your body, get healthier, or become more independent. Make goals that you can actually reach, keep track of your progress, and enjoy your successes along the way. Don't forget that each step you take is one more that makes you healthier and happy.

Getting Past Obstacles to Exercise

Everyone knows that exercise is very important for people with peripheral neuropathy, especially those who also have diabetes. But let's be honest: life can be unpredictable, making it hard to put on your shoes and move. This section will show you how to get around these problems so that nothing gets in the way of you enjoying the many benefits of exercise.

Figuring Out Your Own Obstacles

Knowing what the problem is is the first thing that needs to be done to get past it. Do you have trouble with not having enough time, energy, or motivation?

Maybe you're not moving because you're in pain, afraid of getting hurt, or can't get to the services you need. It's possible that all of these things are to blame. Take a moment to think about your problems and figure out what makes them special. As soon as you know what you're up against, you can make a plan to deal with it.

Getting Through the Time Crunch

One of the main reasons people don't exercise is that they think they don't have time. But don't forget that even short amounts of exercise every day can add up. Instead of trying to work out for an hour at a time, try doing it three times for 20 minutes each. You could go for a quick walk during your lunch break, stretch while watching TV, or park farther away from where you need to go and walk the rest of the way. You'll be amazed at how much these short times of moving around can add up.

How to Get Motivated

There are ways to grow your motivation, even though it can change quickly. Set exciting, attainable goals for yourself and keep track of your progress. No matter how small your accomplishments may seem, you should be proud of them. Find someone to work out with who will push you and keep you honest. You could also join an exercise class or group where you can meet people who have the same goals as you. Remember that exercise should be fun, so find things you are excited about doing.

Making you feel more energetic

Neuropathy often makes people tired, but that doesn't mean you can't reach your exercise goals. Start out slowly and build up the volume and length of your workouts over time. Pick tasks that are right for your level of fitness, and don't be afraid to change exercises if you need to. Break up your workouts into shorter times with rest periods in between if you're feeling tired. Most importantly, make sure you get enough rest and eat well to keep your body going.

How to Deal with Pain and Illness

Talk to your doctor or a physical trainer if pain is stopping you. Their job is to help you make an exercise plan that is safe, efficient, and fits your needs. You can also make a lot of changes to workouts to make them less painful. Say you have trouble walking. Try swimming or water exercises instead. They are low-impact and easy on the joints. Remember that moving around even a little can help ease your pain and make you feel better overall.

Getting Over Your Fears and Anxiety

A real worry for many people with neuropathy is getting hurt or falling. Do something, though. Don't let it stop you. Start with low-impact sports like walking, swimming, or tai chi that are less likely to hurt you. As you get stronger and more confident, slowly make the workout harder. If you're afraid of falling, you could use a cane or walker to help you, or you could work out with a friend or family member who can assist you if required.

Accessible Buildings and Facilities

Not being able to get to a gym or fitness center shouldn't stop you from working out. You can move around at home or outside in many ways. There are a lot of free workout videos and plans online, or you can buy some simple exercise gear, like dumbbells or resistance bands. If you like being outside, check out the parks, trails, and walking tracks in your area. You can even use park chairs, stairs, or other features to make your own circuit workout.

Accepting Help and Community

Don't forget that you don't have to do this by yourself. You should surround yourself with friends, family, and healthcare workers who will be there for you and help you. You might want to join a support group or an online community where you can talk to people who are going through the same things you are. It can be very empowering to share your stories and learn from others.

Happy to see your progress

Don't forget to enjoy your wins in the process. Every little thing you do to become more active is a win. Keep a journal to keep track of your progress. Reward yourself when you hit important goals, and let your support network know about your successes. Don't forget that every little thing counts, and you should be proud of everything you've done.

Getting Past Obstacles to Exercise

We've already talked about how important it is to work out to help with peripheral neuropathy. But let's be honest: life gets busy, and it can be tough to stick to a workout plan. That or you don't know where to begin because you're in pain or tired. Or maybe you're down because of failures or a lack of drive. No matter what is stopping you, remember that you're not alone. There are problems that many people with neuropathy face. If you know how to deal with them, you can get past them and enjoy the benefits of living a busy life.

Common Obstacles and Ways to Get Past Them

Pain is one of the main reasons people don't exercise. It's normal to want to avoid things that might make your neuropathy pain worse if you have it. But studies have shown that exercise can help ease the pain of neuropathy over time. The important thing is to start slowly and build up the volume and length of your workouts over time. If you want to keep your joints healthy, do things like walks, swimming, or yoga. Also, if you feel pain while working out, stop and take a break.

Another usual problem is being tired. Neuropathy can make you feel tired and worn out at times. But did you know that working out can give you more energy? Even though it might not make sense, being active can help your circulation and make you feel more awake and aware. Start with short, low-impact workouts and build up to longer ones as your energy rises.

A physical therapist or certified diabetes instructor can help you figure out where to begin if you don't know what to do. Your wants and limitations will be taken into account when they help you make a personalized exercise plan. As you work to reach your goals, they can also give you advice and help.

Some people don't exercise because they're afraid of falling. Neuropathy can make it harder to keep your balance and move around, which can make you more likely to fall. Keep moving, though, and don't let your fear stop you. Some movements, like tai chi or yoga, can help you get more stable and not fall over. Additionally, you can use aids such as walkers or canes to boost your confidence.

Another common problem is a lack of drive. It can be hard to keep up with a workout plan when you're not wanting to do it. One way to deal with this is to do things you enjoy. If you don't like going to the gym, don't feel like you have to. You can be busy in a lot of different ways, such as by dancing, gardening, or playing with your grandchildren. Find something you're excited about.

Setting goals that you can reach is another good idea.

Do not try to do too much too soon. Set small goals that you can reach at first, and as you get stronger and more confident, raise them. Enjoy the little wins along the way, no matter how small they may seem.

You might also find it helpful to work out with someone or join an exercise class. Working out with a friend can help you stay motivated and give you support. It can also be fun and social.

The Power of Sticking With It

Not all growth happens in a straight line. It's normal to have days when you don't want to work out or when things go wrong. Try not to give up. Things like this happen on every trip. Keeping going is what matters. A little exercise is better than none at all.

One way to stay motivated is to write down your goals and success in a journal. Note how you feel before and after each workout. Write down any changes in your pain, tiredness, or mood. This can help you see how working out is making your life better and motivate you to keep going.

Giving yourself a prize for your hard work is another way to stay on track. Spend some time on yourself after you meet a goal. You could get a massage, read a new book, or go out with friends. This can help strengthen the link between working out and feeling good.

It takes time, patience, and persistence to get past the

things that make it hard to exercise. You can reach your goals and make your life better, though, if you have the right plans and help. Don't forget that training is for more than just your body. It has to do with physical and mental health as well. In addition to making your muscles stronger and your blood flow better, moving your body can also improve your happiness, lower your stress, and make you feel better all around. Let neuropathy not stop you from enjoying the fun and health perks of moving around.

Chapter 8: Coping with the Emotional Impact of Neuropathy

Dealing with Anxiety, Depression, and Sleep Problems

Living with peripheral neuropathy can be very hard on your emotions, and it's normal to feel anxious, depressed, or have trouble sleeping. A lot of the time, these problems are linked and can have a big effect on your health and quality of life. But remember that you are not alone and that there are many good ways to deal with and even get past these mental problems.

Anxiety: For many people, the doubt and pain that come with peripheral neuropathy can make them anxious. It can be very hard to deal with the constant pain, the fear that the condition will get worse, or the thought of how it might affect daily life. There are many things you can do to deal with worry if you are having a hard time with it.

Mindfulness and relaxation exercises, like yoga, meditation, and deep breathing, can help you deal with your worry and feel like you're back in charge. You can focus on the present moment, calm your mind, and let go of stress in your body by doing these things. Another great way to deal with worry is to do a lot of exercise every day.

It makes endorphins, which are natural mood boosts that can help you feel better and less anxious. Doing things you enjoy as hobbies and interests can also help you forget about your problems and give you a sense of purpose and satisfaction.

Depression: Living with chronic pain and possible limits that come with peripheral neuropathy can also make you depressed. Some of the most common signs of depression are sadness, hopelessness, and losing interest in things you used to enjoy. Talking to a mental health professional is very important if you're having these signs. You can get the help and support you need from them to get through this tough time.

Cognitive-behavioral treatment (CBT) is one of the best ways to treat depression. It teaches you how to deal with your feelings and helps you figure out and change the negative thought patterns that make you depressed. Support groups can also be very helpful.

They give you a safe place to talk about your problems, connect with people who understand what you're going through, and get power from how strong they   are.
Not able to sleep: Peripheral neuropathy can cause pain and discomfort that can keep you from sleeping, which can make you tired and unable to concentrate.

Anxiety and sadness can get worse when you don't get enough sleep, making a vicious cycle. There are, however, things you can do to improve the quality of your sleep.

A better night's sleep can be achieved by sticking to a regular sleep schedule, making a relaxing bedtime routine, and making sure your bedroom is cool, dark, and quiet. If pain is keeping you up at night, talk to your doctor about how to deal with it. They might suggest painkillers, physical therapy, or other treatments to help you deal with your pain and sleep better.

The Importance of Self-Care: Taking care of anxiety, depression, and sleep issues needs a comprehensive method that puts self-care first. Eating a healthy diet, working out regularly, learning how to relax, and doing things you enjoy are all important parts of taking care of yourself. Don't forget that taking care of your mental health is just as important as dealing with your neuropathy symptoms.

Looking for Help: Make sure you know that you don't have to go through this alone. Family, friends, or a support group can help you feel better by listening and being open. Don't be afraid to get help from a professional if you're having trouble with anxiety, sadness, or sleep. You can handle these problems better and have a better quality of life with the help of a therapist or counselor.

It can be hard to live with peripheral neuropathy, but it doesn't have to rule your life. You can take charge of your mental health and live a full and satisfying life despite your diagnosis if you deal with your anxiety, depression, and sleep problems. Don't forget that you're not alone and that there is help out there to help you do well.

Building up your resilience and getting help

It can be very hard to deal with your feelings when you have peripheral neuropathy. The pain, numbness, tingling, and weakness that you feel in your body can make you angry, sad, anxious, or even depressed. Even though the road is hard, remember that you're not alone and that you can build the strength to do well despite the problems.

Being resilient means being able to get back on your feet after something bad happens, to deal with change, and to find meaning and purpose in your life. There's no need to ignore or act like the problems don't exist. It means being aware of the problems and pain you're going through while also focused on your resources, strengths, and ability to handle things.

Having a good attitude is one of the most important things you can do to become more resilient. This doesn't mean you have to be happy all the time or hide how you feel. It means noticing the good things in your life, being thankful for them, and trying to see problems in a new way. It means not dwelling on the things you can't change but instead concentrating on the things you can.

Having good ways to deal with problems is another important part of being resilient. These tips can help you deal with your physical issues, feel less stressed, and be healthier overall. Some good ways to deal with stress are:

• Exercise: Being active regularly can help your blood flow, ease pain, and improve your happiness. Make sure you do things that you enjoy and that are safe for you.
• Relaxation techniques: Deep breathing, yoga, and meditation are all activities that can help you feel less stressed, sleep better, and relax.

• CBT (cognitive behavioral therapy): This kind of treatment can help you figure out and change harmful ways of thinking, as well as learn better ways to deal with stress and handle your feelings.

• Mindfulness: Being mindful means focusing on the present moment without judging it. It can help you understand your feelings and thoughts better, lower your stress, and make you healthier.

• Creative expression: Doing creative things like dancing, making art, writing, or playing music can help you deal with stress and show how you feel.

Getting stronger is not something you can do by yourself. Making friends with people who get what you're going through is important. People in this group could be family, friends, support groups, or online organizations. Sharing your feelings, getting help, and learning from other people can be very powerful.

For people with peripheral neuropathy, support groups can be very helpful. They give people a safe place to talk about their problems, learn from others' experiences, and get mental support. You can find support groups online or in your neighborhood.

It's also important to get help from a professional if neuropathy is making it hard for you to deal with your emotions. A therapist or counselor can help you learn how to deal with problems, handle your feelings, and feel better in general. They can also help you figure out if there are any deeper problems that are making you feel bad.

Living with peripheral neuropathy is a process, not a place you get to. It's a trip that needs strength, persistence, and help. But the trip can also help you grow as a person, learn more about yourself, and appreciate life more.

Don't forget that you have friends and family. You can build your endurance and find support through a lot of different channels. Even though peripheral neuropathy can be hard, you can do well if you take care of yourself, connect with other people, and get skilled help when you need it.

Getting to Know Other People: Online Communities and Support Groups

Sometimes having peripheral neuropathy makes life feel like a fight. The tingling, numbness, and pain can be too much to handle, and the mental effects can be just as hard. It's easy to feel like no one else gets what you're going through and cut off from the world. You're not alone, though. Millions of people around the world have peripheral neuropathy, and many have found comfort and strength in talking to other people who   understand.

Support groups can help you find your tribe.

For people with peripheral neuropathy, support groups can be very helpful. When you join one of these groups, you can feel safe and comfortable talking about your problems and get helpful advice from people who are also facing the same problems. Support groups can be found in a lot of places, like hospitals, community centers, and even online.

Giving people a sense of community is one of the best things about support groups. Connecting with people who understand your problems can help you deal with the loneliness that comes with having a long-term illness like peripheral neuropathy. It can be very motivating to know that you are not alone on your journey.

Support groups can also help you with your emotions and give you a lot of useful knowledge. Members can help each other deal with their problems, give each other tips on how to use the healthcare system, and just listen when you need to. A lot of support groups also have outside speakers, like doctors, therapists, and nutritionists, who talk about different parts of living with peripheral neuropathy.

What Online Communities Can Do for You

For people with peripheral neuropathy, internet communities have become very helpful in this day and age. You can find these groups on online boards, social media sites, and specialized websites. They make it easy to connect with others, talk about your experiences, get help and information, and connect with others.

Many of the benefits of face-to-face support groups are also available in online communities. The main differences are that online communities are easier to join and anonymous. No matter what time of day or night it is, you can connect with other people from your own home. You can join online discussions without giving away your name if you'd rather stay anonymous.

There is a lot of knowledge about peripheral neuropathy in a lot of online communities. This includes articles, blog posts, and new research. You can also join groups and chat rooms to talk to other people and share your thoughts. In some places, you can even join a virtual support group and talk to other people through voice or video chat.

Getting Started

There are some things you should think about if you want to join an online club or support group. First, look into groups and pick one that feels right to you. There are lots of different kinds of groups, and each has its own purpose and vibe. Some groups may be more about giving emotional support, while others may be more about giving knowledge.

When you find a group, be sure to say hello and get to know the other people in it. Talk about your problems, ask questions, and help other people. Always keep in mind that support groups work both ways. You can build a strong and long-lasting sense of community by helping each other out.

Getting in touch with people who understand your problems can be life-changing. You may feel less alone, more in control, and better able to deal with the problems that come with peripheral neuropathy. There are clear benefits to connecting with others, whether you choose to do so in a real-life support group or an online community.

Reach out to other people. You might be shocked at how much it can help you live a better life with peripheral neuropathy.

Chapter 9: Advocating for Your Health: Tips for Effective Communication

Talking to Your Healthcare Team
It can be hard to live with peripheral neuropathy caused by diabetes, but know that you're not alone. Your healthcare team is your loyal friend and is dedicated to giving you the best care and support they can. To effectively manage your peripheral neuropathy and reach your best level of health, you must communicate openly and honestly with your healthcare team.

How to Work Together with Your Healthcare Team

Your healthcare team is like a health partner for you. Everyone on the team, from your general care doctor and neurologist to your diabetes educator and physical therapist, brings something different to the table. You and your partner can work together to make a personalized care plan that fits your wants and goals. Remember that you know the most about your body and what it's going through. Your health care team is there to help, listen, and give you advice.

Getting Ready for Your Meetings

You can have more useful and helpful talks with your healthcare team if you prepare ahead of time. Write down any questions or worries you may have before your appointments. It might help to write down your symptoms and any changes or trends you notice in a journal. Keep track of your progress and let your healthcare team know about any changes you make to your lifestyle or try a new therapy. This information will help them figure out what's wrong with you and make a care plan that fits your needs.

Talking about your symptoms and worries Of course

It is very important that you describe your symptoms correctly and clearly so that your healthcare team can understand what you are going through with peripheral neuropathy. When you talk about your symptoms, be as detailed as you can. Instead of saying "My feet feel weird," you could say "My feet feel numb and tingly, like pins and needles." If your symptoms come and go, describe when they do, how long they last, and what makes them happen. If you don't understand something your healthcare provider says, don't be afraid to ask them to explain it to you. You can also ask them to say something again or explain it in a different way.

Taking an active role in your care

Remember that you are in charge of your health care. Ask questions, find out more, and say what you want in terms of your care to be an active participant. Talk to your healthcare team about alternative therapies or complementary techniques if you're interested in trying them. You can compare the possible pros and cons and decide what the best thing to do is. If you're having trouble controlling your peripheral neuropathy, be open and honest about it. Your healthcare team can help you get past problems and reach your goals by giving you support and useful tools.

How to Have Difficult Conversations

When you talk to your healthcare team, you may sometimes talk about personal or hard subjects. Don't forget that they are there to help you and want to hear your worries. Do not be afraid to talk about how you feel if you are stressed or upset. Your healthcare team can understand, reassure, and help you. Don't be afraid to say something if you're not happy with some part of your care. You can find solutions that meet your wants and expectations if you work together.

Making Friends and Building Trust

Respect, open conversation, and making decisions together are the building blocks of a strong, trusting relationship with your healthcare team. Spend some time getting to know the people who are taking care of you. Tell us about yourself, your goals, and your fears. Don't forget that they are people too, and they care about your well-being. You can even ask them about working with people who have peripheral neuropathy if you feel safe doing so. This can help you learn more about your situation and the different ways you can treat it.

Staying Informed and Giving People Power

It's true that knowledge is power. You can be an active advocate for your health if you know about peripheral neuropathy and how to treat it. Ask your health care team for suggestions on good books, blogs, and support groups. Go to classes or seminars that teach you about diabetes and peripheral neuropathy. Being able to make smart choices about your care and take charge of your own health will depend on how much you know.

Having a party for your wins

Taking care of peripheral neuropathy is an ongoing process, so don't forget to enjoy the small wins along the way. Every win is worth celebrating, whether it's better control of your blood sugar, a new therapy that works for you, or just feeling more sure of your ability to handle your condition. Share your health care team's accomplishments and let them know how much you value their help. Don't forget that you're not on this trip by yourself. You can do well with peripheral neuropathy and live a full, busy life if you talk to your healthcare team, take part, and build a strong relationship with them.

How to Get Around the Healthcare System

It can be hard to live with peripheral neuropathy, especially if it is caused by diabetes. You are not alone, though. Knowing how to use the healthcare system to get the care you need is an important part of taking care of your situation. You will be able to make smart choices about your health and be an active part of your care.

Putting together your healthcare team

Take care of your peripheral neuropathy as a group effort. You, as captain, are the leader of this team and make the plays. Your general care doctor, a neurologist who specializes in peripheral neuropathy, a podiatrist who takes care of your feet, an endocrinologist who manages your diabetes, and maybe even a pain specialist or a physical therapist are all around you. Each of these workers has a special skill that can help you deal with different parts of your condition. It's important to get along with your healthcare team. Tell your doctor the truth about your symptoms, worries, and any changes in your health. Remember that they are not just experts telling you what to do for treatment; they are your partners in taking care of your health. Being involved in your own care can make a big difference in how well you do.

Learning About Your Treatment Options

There is no one way to treat peripheral neuropathy that works for everyone. Your healthcare team will make a treatment plan for you based on your symptoms, health background, and way of life. Some of the things that may be used are painkillers, treatments like physical therapy or transcutaneous electrical nerve stimulation (TENS), and changes to the person's diet and exercise routine.

It's important to know what treatment choices you have. Find out what the pros and cons of each treatment are, how they will affect your everyday life, and what results you can expect. If something isn't clear, don't be afraid to ask for more information. Don't forget that the goal is to find a treatment plan that fits your life perfectly and works best for you.

Why self-advocacy is important

Being a self-advocate means taking charge of your health and well-being. It means standing up for your needs, asking questions, and looking for the help and knowledge you need to deal with your condition well. You should not be afraid to get a second opinion if you are not sure about a diagnosis or treatment plan. Being ready for your meetings is another part of self-advocacy. Write down your symptoms, including how bad they are and how often they happen, as well as any vitamins or medicines you're taking and any questions you have for your doctor. This can give your doctor a better idea of what's wrong with you and help them decide how to treat you.

How to Understand Insurance and Costs

It can be expensive to take care of a long-term disease like peripheral neuropathy. It is important to know what your insurance covers and what costs you may have to pay out of pocket. Don't be afraid to call your insurance company to find out what they cover and what tools are available to help you deal with your condition.

People with diabetes and peripheral neuropathy can get cash help from a lot of different groups. Your healthcare team can help you find these places and fill out the forms to get help. Remember that taking care of your health shouldn't cost you a lot of money. There are things that can be used to assist.

Taking Charge of Your Health

It can be hard to deal with peripheral neuropathy, but know that you are not alone. The healthcare system can be hard to understand, but you can take charge of your health if you have the right healthcare team, know what treatments are available to you, and are good at speaking up for yourself.

Don't forget that this trip is about more than just taking care of a condition. It's about making your life better and surviving even though you have peripheral neuropathy. You can achieve the best health and well-being by being involved in your care and speaking up for your needs.

Finding Resources and Help with Money

It can be hard to find your way around when you have peripheral neuropathy and diabetes at the same time. You're not alone on this journey, though. There are a lot of tools and possible financial aid programs out there that can help you deal with your condition and make your life better. Let's look at these choices together and figure out how you can get the help you need.

Using Resources in the Community

The people in your area can be a great source of help. People who have peripheral neuropathy can get help from a lot of groups, both big and small. Some of these are educational workshops, support groups, exercise classes designed just for people with neuropathy, and even clinics that make shoes for people with neuropathy. First, get in touch with the diabetes association or neighborhood health center in your area.

A lot of the time, they can help you find programs and services in your area that will help you. Always keep in mind that support groups are very helpful. Getting in touch with people who are going through similar problems can be very comforting and energizing. It can make a huge difference to share stories, ways to deal with problems, and words of support.

Governmental groups: your allies

On a national level, groups like the American Diabetes Association and the Foundation for Peripheral Neuropathy are very helpful. They have a lot of useful information, like the newest study results, treatment options, and tips for taking care of yourself. On many of their websites, there are online groups where people with neuropathy can meet and talk with each other from all over the country.

These groups also work to get laws passed that help people with neuropathy and diabetes. Staying up to date on their plans will help you be a strong voice for your own health.

How to Find Financial Help: Getting Around

Taking care of peripheral neuropathy can be hard when it comes to money. Medications, therapies, special shoes, and gadgets that help can all add up. Remember, though, that you don't have to carry this weight by yourself.

There are several ways to get cash help. Companies that make medicines often have plans to help patients who qualify. Medicare and Medicaid may help pay some of your costs. Depending on your policy, private insurance may also cover some of your costs. You should call your insurance company to fully understand your benefits.

People with long-term conditions like neuropathy can sometimes get grants or other cash help from non-profits. Some hospitals and clinics also have social workers who can help you look into your choices for getting financial help. Don't be afraid to ask for help; it's the first thing that will help you get the things you need.

Getting behind clinical trials and research

We are always learning more about peripheral neuropathy and diabetes through research. People who take part in clinical trials can get cutting-edge treatments before they are widely offered. Being a part of a trial can be a way to get expert care for little or no cost while also helping to learn more about medicine.

Talk to your doctor about clinical studies if you're interested. They can help you figure out which trials are right for you and walk you through the process.

Information that gives people power

One of the best ways to fight for your health is to empower yourself with information. Take the time to learn as much as you can about your situation. Learn about the different kinds of neuropathy, how to treat them, and the newest study results. What you know will help you feel more sure in the choices you make about your care.

You should remember that it can take a while to find tools and money to help you. If you can't find everything you need right away, don't give up. It pays off to keep going. Keep looking into your choices, asking questions, and getting in touch with groups.

Remember that you have help available and that you are not alone. You can do well even if you have peripheral neuropathy if you have the right tools and a strong will.

Conclusion: Living Your Best Life with Peripheral Neuropathy: A Message of Hope

You can still live a normal life even though you have peripheral neuropathy. It might mean making changes to your habits and way of life, but it doesn't have to mean giving up happiness, satisfaction, and a life well lived. Not only do many people with peripheral neuropathy deal with their condition, they also thrive, discovering new interests, growing in their relationships, and making the most of every day.

You're not alone.

Don't forget that you're not on this trip by yourself. There are millions of people living with peripheral neuropathy around the world, and there are a huge number of tools, support groups, and communities that can help, understand, and cheer them on. Don't be afraid to talk about your feelings with your healthcare team, your friends and family, or online groups where people can relate.

The Strength of Being Positive and Strong

Studies have shown that people with chronic conditions like peripheral neuropathy can greatly improve their quality of life by having a good attitude and being strong. Focusing on what you can control, taking on new tasks, and celebrating small wins can help you feel hopeful and in charge, which will help you deal with the ups and downs of having this condition.

Why self-care is important

People who have peripheral neuropathy need to make self-care a priority. This includes taking care of your mental and emotional health as well as your physical issues through therapies, medications, and changes to your lifestyle. Do things that make you happy, spend time with people you care about, learn how to relax, and if you need to, get professional help.

Keeping busy and active

Keeping up an active lifestyle is important for controlling peripheral neuropathy and improving health in general. Regular exercise can help your happiness, lower your pain, and improve your circulation. If you find traditional types of exercise hard, there are lots of low-impact things you can do that you can still enjoy, like yoga, walking, or swimming. Keeping your mind active with hobbies, social activities, or volunteer work can also help avoid depression and anxiety and give you a sense of purpose.

What role do education and advocacy play?

Knowing more about peripheral neuropathy can help you make choices about your care that are best for you and speak up for your needs. Keep up with the newest studies, treatment options, and support services that are out there. Don't be afraid to ask questions, get second views, and, if it makes sense, take part in clinical trials. Speaking up for yourself and other people who have peripheral neuropathy can help millions of people learn about the condition and make their lives better.

A Hopeful Look at the Future

Even though peripheral neuropathy doesn't have a cure yet, study is still going on and new treatments are always being made. You can keep your hope alive for a future with better treatment options and maybe even a cure by staying up to date on the latest research.

Stay in mind that having peripheral neuropathy does not mean you will always have it. It's hard, but it's also a chance to learn how to be stronger and find new meaning in life. You can live your best life even if you have peripheral neuropathy if you think positively, take care of yourself, stay busy and involved, and learn new things.